SHARING

LIVES

A Tale of Two Kidneys

Rebecca S. Carlisle

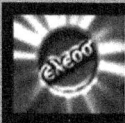

Eleos Press

Rogersville, AL

First Edition
Sharing Lives

Author: Rebecca S. Carlisle
ISBN-13: 978-0692247020

Cover Design: Eleos Press www.eleospress.com
Interior Formatting: Eleos Press www.eleospress.com

Also available in eBook form

PRINTED IN THE UNITED STATES OF AMERICA

Proceeds from the sale of this book will be donated to the Mason Transplant Center at Piedmont Hospital in Atlanta, Georgia

This book is dedicated to our sister-in-law, Sheila Carlisle, with love and gratitude.

TABLE OF CONTENTS

Acknowledgments

Special thanks to my family and friends for their support and encouragement in the writing of this book:

Sam Carlisle Barham
Richard Carlisle
Shea Carlisle
Linda Petry
Cheryl Pollard
Leanne Whitehead

A special recognition also goes out to the following people:

Edward Fredrickson, MD
Erica Hartman, MD
Hospital Staff at Piedmont Hospital,
Miami Valley Hospital
Tom Scouller, NP
Ann Taylor, Coordinator
Erik Weise, MD
Leanne Whitehead, Coordinator
Joshua Wolfe, MD
Carlos Zayas, MD

Introduction

"It was the best of times, it was the worst of times, it was the age of wisdom, it was the age of foolishness, it was the epoch of belief, it was the epoch of incredulity, it was the season of Light, it was the season of Darkness, it was the season of hope, it was the winter of despair, we had everything before us, we had nothing before us, we were all going to Heaven, we were all going direct the other way . . ." (A Tale of Two Cities, Charles Dickens, 1859)

Wait just one moment…while it may be Charles Dickens' story let me tell you a story just as remarkable. While I admire Charles Dickens as a great writer, his story was fiction. There are very few similarities between the book of Charles Dickens and this book. Sharing Lives: A Tale of Two Kidneys is a compilation of true stories of ordinary people, both young and old, who gave unselfishly to those they loved so they could live.

i

It is a story of a young girl who received a kidney more than thirty years ago. She has lived a very rewarding life with three children and seven beautiful grandchildren. All was made possible because a family gave a kidney to her during their time of grief. A story of a young mother who gave her kidney to her mother without a second thought to her own life just because she trusted and loved God knowing He would bless her and her family. Then there is my story of two couples matched to give their kidneys to someone they had never met, so a person they loved could receive a kidney. A match made possible through the Paired Donor program. A hospital which worked with another hospital to make it happen. The miracles made possible through the love of God and His blessings on the people involved.

Part 1: From the Ashes of Grief Comes a New Beginning

Chapter 1 The Accident

The morning started early, with her rising at five and leaving by six. Monday mornings were always hectic after a busy weekend. She had just finished her freshman year in college at UAB, University of Alabama in Birmingham, majoring in elementary education. She always wanted to be a teacher for as long as she could remember. Teaching was a way to help others. The previous year she had graduated from high school with honors. Her family was so proud of her. She was their only daughter with two younger brothers. During the summer she decided to live at home and work at the public swimming pool as a lifeguard in Childersburg. Fall semester would begin in a few weeks and she was saving her summer money to help cover the cost of books and supplies. She had received scholarships when she graduated, but college was costing more than she had anticipated. She wanted to ease the burden of her parents paying for everything the scholarships did not cover.

She especially loved the summer months with the warm weather. She and her family had just come back from a trip to Gulf Shores. Her face was pink with a glow from a little too much sun. Today she was looking forward to meeting

3

up with friends to celebrate her nineteenth birthday. She had met a boy while away at college, but she was not interested in getting serious. She had too much to do before even thinking about marriage.

She enjoyed singing and going to the church she had attended for as long as she could remember. When she was at home,she played the piano for Sunday school. Life was good and she was looking forward to another year at UAB with plans to transfer to the University of Alabama in Tuscaloosa during her junior year. Both her parents had been graduates of the university and she wanted to follow in their footsteps. Today she was going to volunteer at Vacation Bible School (VBS). This was her third year volunteering at VBS where she enjoyed working with the children. She kissed her mom and dad goodbye, telling them she loved them and out the door she ran.

Her parents had surprised her with a car for graduation. It was the perfect gift and she needed a car which did not stay in the repair shop all the time. Her dad wanted her to have a safe, practical car that was good on gas.

Traffic was especially busy even for a Monday morning. Everyone was returning to work after being off the week before for the Independence Day Celebration. She turned on the radio to her favorite station. She lived about five miles from Highway I-20. It had been raining earlier that morning and the roads were wet. The sun was beginning to come up over the horizon. Feeling great with the whole world at her fingertips, she entered the ramp onto I-20 heading toward Birmingham. There was some traffic, but she was moving along at a steady speed.

All of a sudden, without any warning, a car from the oncoming lane was barreling toward her, out of control. The two cars hit head on. The impact could be heard for miles. Paramedics would report the accident as one of the worst they had ever seen. Her car was so badly mangled, they could not tell the make or model. The car that hit her was a minivan with a mother and father and a five-year-old child. They were killed on impact. In the crumpled wreck of metal they found her unconscious, but breathing. She needed immediate medical attention. The paramedics transported her to UAB Hospital in Birmingham. They worked with her all the way to the hospital trying to keep her alive. When she arrived, the doctors worked quickly checking her vital signs.

Tests would reveal the impact was life threatening. Her brain was hemorrhaging. She was bleeding between the brain and the layer of membrane which covered the brain. She was placed on a ventilator to assist her breathing. Her parents were notified and they rushed to her side. Her mother collapsed when she received the news from the doctors. The tests indicated there were no brain waves. She just could not accept the news her only daughter was dead. They had been so close and in an instant she was gone. All her hopes and dreams were now a thing of the past. She did not think she could go on without her. Her daughter would never be a wife or mother. She wouldn't grow old and experience the joys of being a grandmother.

The doctors discussed with them about donating her organs, but her mother was so upset not wanting to discuss it with the doctors. They were taken to her room to spend some time alone with her. The mother could not stand the thought of losing her daughter and now they wanted to use her organs. How dare the hospital come to her after she had lost the most precious thing in her life? The grief was unbearable. It was hard to imagine she was no longer here with them.

When they entered the room and saw her on a ventilator, they knew in their hearts what they needed to do. She was lying there so calmly and peacefully. She looked so petite and angelic as if she was sleeping.

They had worshiped in church as a family and had a strong belief in God. As they prayed together, a peace came upon them. They knew she would have wanted to help others even in death. Her parents notified the doctors of their wishes to donate her organs.

Chapter 2 Special Gift for Linda

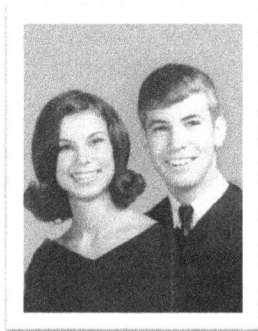

Aubin, Linda's husband, was an early riser. This morning was no different and he would get up quietly so he would not wake her. They had three small children and Linda was on dialysis which tended to make her tire more easily. Aubin did not hear the phone ring that morning so Linda, sleepy, got out of bed to answer it. It was the call she had been anxiously waiting for, but now she was not sure she was ready for it.

It was Dr. Whelchel's office in Birmingham, Alabama. All she heard was they had a kidney for her. The rest of the conversation seemed to move in slow motion as they gave her instructions. She could not wait to tell Aubin. He quickly got ready and went to his store to tell Christine, his assistant, the news, and see if she would open up.

Linda called Aubin's parents who were so excited and came immediately. They had hoped for this moment to arrive as much as Linda.

9

Rebecca S. Carlisle

Mary Lynn, Aubin's sister, had planned to come and care for the children so her parents could go to the hospital when Linda had surgery. Linda's excitement of getting a kidney was almost too much to comprehend. She tried to stay calm and convince Aubin's parents there was no need to hurry, but deep down inside she wanted to get to the hospital as fast as possible. Linda called her parents to give them the wonderful news. It was certainly an answer to their prayers.

Linda quickly got dressed and decided to wake her children. Six-year-old Robin, her daughter, was so sleepy she didn't realize what her mother was saying, Linda kissed her, and told her to go back to sleep. Five seconds after the door closed Robin was standing in the doorway with a big smile. Linda went upstairs to tell the boys. Her sons, eleven-year-old Clay and eight-year-old Chris, jumped out of bed and began their own plan of action. They had known this day would come and they were ready for it.

Before leaving, Linda called Jane, her sister. Jane's birthday was two days away and she started crying knowing this was the best birthday present ever.

The goodbyes were loving, and filled with apprehension. Linda didn't know how long it would be before she could see her children after surgery. One thing she did not have to worry about was her children. They were in great

10

hands. Linda had not been able to care for them the way she wanted for the past year. In fact, they had been taking care of her.

Chapter 3 Trip to the Hospital

It was a two-hour drive from home to UAB Hospital in Birmingham, Alabama. On the way Aubin and Linda talked calmly trying not to discuss the surgery. As they drove listening to the radio, they began to hear about an accident and death reports. As they listened they both wondered if they had just heard about the donor. Through all the excitement Linda had not thought about the kidney donor. It dawned on her this kidney had come from someone who had just died. She quietly said a prayer for the family. She thanked God for the special gift she was receiving and she asked God to be with her family and the family of the one who gave her this gift of life.

Chapter 4 Preparing for Surgery

Dr. Whelchel and Dr. Luke came into the room smiling from ear to ear. Dr. Whelchel had told Linda earlier he would find a kidney, but she had no idea it would be so soon.

The doctors informed her that the kidney would come from a nineteen-year-old female.

They began prepping Linda for surgery. The first thing was for Linda to have a dialysis treatment for three hours.

Linda's mother and father came into the Dialysis Unit. Her daddy had never seen her on the machine. The news of a new kidney had made him cry, but since then he could not quit smiling. As the three hours passed on the dialysis machine, Linda wondered if this would be her last time.

Chapter 5 Dialysis Treatments

Dialysis had been the most traumatic experience of her life. If it had not been for Dr. Rankin, her Nephrologist, and her family, she might not have been able to handle dialysis treatments.

January through March had been the worst. She vomited each time and would collapse for a day and a half after each treatment. At first dialysis was twice a week for three-and-a-half hours and increased to three times a week for three hours. She was finally able to tolerate the treatments, but was unable to do much more, especially take care of her family.

She had lost thirty pounds and she did not have the energy to manage her household. Dialysis treatments zapped her of all her strength and energy. Caring for her three children and a husband was something she always enjoyed, but she could no longer keep up with the demands. She found not being able to take care of them was heartbreaking. Everyone chipped in and they did not seem to mind helping her.

Chapter 6 Preparing for a Transplant

Dr. Rankin convinced Linda that Birmingham was the best place to have a transplant. Dialysis was not the best answer for someone who had a chance at a better life. She had gone to Birmingham the previous April for an evaluation. Linda and her mother had the same blood type and it appeared her mother would be a donor for her. Linda and her mother were scheduled for a live donor transplant two weeks prior. Everything looked good until the last cross match the day before surgery. The last test was positive on the cross match and they were sent home very disappointed. Her father had been rejected as a donor in December. Her two sisters and brother were tested, but they were not matches. They were heart broken when they did not match. It appeared she would have to wait on a cadaver.

Chapter 7 The Kidney Transplant

Aubin was sitting with Linda while they were waiting for the stretcher. Linda was shaking uncontrollably so Aubin held her and tried to calm her. He knew she was scared and he wanted to be brave for her, but he was also scared. Dr. Rivas explained the spinal injection would help to calm her. Dr. Whelchel said the final cross match was negative and they would be able to proceed with the transplant. Wearing his cowboy boots and with country music playing in the background, he began the operation. Linda remembered the sensation of being cut on the right side, but there was no pain. She drifted off and woke up in ICU.

Her hand went to the right side of her abdomen. It was taped and she had no feeling in her legs because of the spinal injection. There were tubes in her hand, neck and nose. Her mouth was dry and the catheter was uncomfortable.

A moment later she realized what had happened. She had a kidney transplant! Did it work? Had it been successful? She called out to the nurse. "Is the kidney working?" The nurse lifted the full bag and said, "It looks like it's working to me." They both smiled and Linda gave a sigh of relief.

Chapter 8 After the Transplant

She said a little prayer and braced herself for the next critical days. She knew rejection would have to be dealt with over the next few weeks. Dr. Whelchel had explained mild rejection could be treated. The antirejection drugs Prednisone and Imuran would help to guard her body against rejecting the new kidney. She began the medicine right away dreading the side effects she had remembered when she had last taken the medication. Immediately she began to feel better. Even after surgery she had more energy than she had in four years.

Chapter 9 The Hospital Stay and Other Transplant Patients

On the fourth day after surgery, Linda's kidney was working as it should—showing no signs of rejection. She could touch her toes and her vital signs were super. During her hospital stay she met so many people just like her. The stories were as individual as the people. Each one with a unique story.

Mrs. Baskin received her transplant the same day as Linda. On the eleventh day her second attempt in four years with a new kidney had failed. They were going to remove the kidney. Linda cried for her and she feared the same thing could happen to her. Linda had talked with Mrs. Baskin earlier and she said she could go back on dialysis without a problem. Mrs. Baskin was grateful for a very happy family life. Linda felt she would be just fine.

She was encouraged by a man she met on her eleventh day after receiving her kidney. He was about to receive his second transplant from a relative. The first kidney transplant had lasted seven years and had slowly quit working. He did not have to be dialyzed after receiving his new kidney. The kidney was working fine.

On the twelfth day in the hospital Julie, a transplant patient Linda had met in April, was going home. She was twenty-two, and this was her third kidney from a relative. She received her first kidney when she was nine. The drugs stunted her growth. Linda met her in April when they were evaluated at the same time. Julie had looked bad and she was very sick. After surgery she had a big smile on her face and she was glowing. She looked like a different person. She said this kidney was going to last forever.

On the thirteenth day Linda was able to leave the hospital for four hours. Aubin brought the children and they went out to eat and to the zoo. She became hot and tired, but enjoyed being with them so much. It was a special day for everyone. Since Linda had been in the hospital, the children seem to have grown some. They wanted to take their mother home. She was homesick and she fought back tears when they left. She wanted to go home, but she was a little scared to be on her own without the safety of the doctors and the constant blood work. The fear of losing the kidney was fresh on her mind.

On the fourteenth day Mary Ellen Baker moved into the room next to Linda. They enjoyed talking and had so much in common. They were both young mothers with loving and supportive husbands. They vowed to always stay in touch.

The Tale of Two Kidneys

Another patient, Jimmy Collins, was blind, and he received his transplant the same day as Linda. They walked twice a day and he was a good companion. He had been through so much in the past year. He had a heart bypass operation after starting dialysis. He was a diabetic and now he had a new kidney. Linda admired his strength. He told her he had to be strong for his children.

Linda made friends with three other young mothers on the floor. They would talk, walk and laugh together. She brought four jumpsuits in different colors which they would wear going up and down the hall. It is great realizing they could once again function as healthy people. All the transplant patients agreed it had been a life changing experience. Everyone was so elated just realizing they could do all the things they did before they got sick.

Chapter 10 Going Home

On the nineteenth day, Linda was released from the hospital to go home. It had been three short weeks. She would be the first kidney transplant patient released from UAB Hospital to go home so soon after the transplant and she was ready. Her kidney function was great and she was tolerating the rejection medication. Dr. Whelchel was pleased with her progress. Dr. Rankin would closely monitor Linda after she left the hospital. She would continue to have blood drawn three times a week and watch for symptoms of rejection. Linda looked forward to doing the simple things she had taken for granted. She looked forward to living each day to its fullest. Linda thanked God for her new life and hoped she would be worthy of His blessings.

Chapter 11 Kidney Rejection

At the end of the fourth week Linda was showing signs of kidney rejection. Dr. Rankin was able to treat her without having to put her in the hospital. The increased dosage of medicine, however limited her already weakened immune system so much that she contracted the CMV virus.[1] The virus is common in the U.S. It rarely causes health problems, except for transplant recipients which have impaired immune systems. The drugs made her very nervous and caused her face to swell. Her face and back broke out in terrible sores. Her hair began to thin and what hair remained was dry and brittle. Her knees hurt when she walked for short periods. She was skinny, but her face looked like a chipmunk. She spent a week in isolation at the hospital in Carrollton and another two weeks in UAB Hospital. She continued to experience side effects from the medication. She did not dwell on this,

---

[1] CMV, which stands for Cytomegalovirus, is a type of herpes virus. 50% to 80% of the people in the United Stated have had a CMV infection by the time they are forty years old, according to the Center for Disease Control. CMV is rarely serious. (http://health.ny.gov April, 2014)

knowing the symptoms would eventually go away.

The hardest thing to deal with during this time was fear. Fear of losing her kidney; fear of being sick again; fear of losing what she had been given. Living one day at a time now seemed impossible. She wanted the wonderful feeling she had after returning home from the hospital after the transplant. It all seemed to be slipping away. It began to show on Aubin's face too. He looked tired and worried. They had looked forward to Linda's recovery and now it was just a great disappointment. It looked like a setback.

During this hard time Dr. Rankin was there for her. Linda was determined to first rid herself of the anxiety and then the virus. It is amazing how much better she began to feel when she turned her fear and frustration over to God. She realized the only control she had over her life was positive thinking and acceptance of whatever lay ahead; with the faith, she would not be alone.

Three weeks after she left the hospital the fever was gone and her strength was returning.

Chapter 12 Sixth Month Anniversary

Linda's sixth month anniversary had arrived and with it a time for celebration. Her numbers were once again super.[2] She enjoyed the best Christmas in six years. Her face was still swollen, but the other symptoms were subsiding. She was feeling normal and she believed she could handle her life once again. She was thankful for her life and the trials along the way which made her realize the importance of living one day at a time.

---

[2] Numbers refers to the tests given to determine kidney function and rejection of the new kidney.Urine tests are used to determine how the kidneys are functioning. (www.nih.gov (May, 2014)

Chapter 13 Against All Odds

It had been twenty years since she received her kidney and there was reason to celebrate another milestone. When Linda received her kidney in 1983, the drugs used were not as successful as the ones used today. Her prospects for survival were at best seven years. There were not that many transplanted kidney success stories. All she asked of God was to let her live long enough to raise her children. God had greater plans for her. Twenty years after receiving her new kidney her children were grown and on their own. Linda and Aubin were enjoying the life of being grandparents.

She was now fifty-three years old and had forgotten what it was like to be so sick. Her kidney function was good and life was absolutely normal.

Her friend, inspiration and life saver Dr. Rankin retired. She would still see him around town and they would hug and reminisce. Dr. Orig took over Linda's health care and she was amazed at Linda's success.

Dr. Whelchel moved from Birmingham to Atlanta. Linda saw him in 1993 at Emory Hospital. He recognized her and called her by name. He had been keeping up with her process through Dr. Rankin.

Mary Ellen and Linda kept in touch for several years. Mary Ellen lost her kidney and had to return to dialysis. She was unable to tolerate the drugs. She was healthy on dialysis the first time and could be again. They quit calling and writing each other. It was hard for Linda to keep telling her how wonderful she was doing knowing Mary Ellen was not doing as well.

Linda and Jimmy corresponded with each other for a few years. He quit responding and she never knew what happened to him.

Out of the three young mothers together in the hospital with Linda one returned to dialysis, one died, she never heard from the other one. Linda was the only one who was continuing to do well.

Both of Aubin's parents died. Linda's parents were in their eighties and both remained lively and well.

Linda was so thankful for Aubin. He was the greatest thing that ever happened to her. Each day she is grateful to be growing older with him.

God had granted her more than she ever thought possible with too many blessings to count. God gave her the joy of raising her children and grandchildren. Linda's oldest grandson, Brennon, told her he knew why God let her live so long. "It's because you help everybody." Everyone who knows Linda will agree she has lived her life to be a blessing to others.

Chapter 14 Thirtieth Anniversary

Linda has reached another milestone and amazed the doctors. She continues to be well and active. Aubin's health is failing him and he was diagnosed with bladder cancer. Linda cares for him as he did for her. She loves him and she is thankful for all he did for her when she was sick.

The date is July 11, 2013 and Linda is living proof of God's love and what He can do for those who love and honor Him. The kidney saved a young mother with three children. No one knew the kidney would last thirty years. A gift of life given, because a nineteen-year-old female loved people and cared for them. She made a difference even in death. Linda often thinks of the girl's family who gave something so precious even though their hearts were breaking. Linda reflects back to all the blessings and memories she has cherished over the years. The young mother is now a beautiful active grandmother with seven grandchildren. She is living the life of her dreams.

Linda often recalls the night she realized she might die. She was a Christian and knew she would be fine, but she had small children. She asked God to allow her to stay with them until they were a little older. At that point she could feel God smiling and saying, "Sweetheart, you will not only raise your children, but you will be there to help raise and enjoy your grandchildren!"

Chapter 15   Life Thirty Years after the Transplant

Five years after the kidney transplant, Aubin and Linda moved to the farm in Ephesus, Georgia. It is where they belonged. It is where they put down roots and made memories. It is where her children found their futures and a place where all her grandkids come to visit.   It's Pawpaw and Nina's house. Chris and Robin built their homes, and live with their families on the Cumbie Farm. A place where they live, love and support each other.

Clay and Stefanie have a son named Colbey Clay. Colbey Clay was the same age as Clay, his dad, when Linda received the kidney thirty years ago.

They moved when they married, but they come to visit.

Chris and Tamantha were married and gave Linda another granddaughter named Hope.

Robin and Tim Meacham have given her five grandchildren, four grandsons, Brennon,

Caden, Luke and Seth and one granddaughter, Caylee Jane. They live on the farm behind Chris.

Aubin's cancer has not returned since his last surgery in 2011. He is slowing down and enjoying life with Linda, his children and grandchildren.

She was a young woman in 1983 only thirty-three years old. Today she is in her sixties. Ask her where those thirty years went and she will tell you she remembers each precious year.

Family is the most important thing to her. Her daddy in his eighties recently said "They were a family connected by prayer." As she watches her parents grow older she is reminded we have a very short time to live the right way and to help those around us.

Linda's legacy will be to help those who need her and to make long-lasting memories for those she loves.

Her kidney function has declined some over the years, but she knows God will take care of her.

The Tale of Two Kidneys

God has granted her more than she asked. Her prayers are to continue to be worthy of what she has received.

This is not the end of her story, just all *for now*. She continues to live each day knowing God has blessed her.

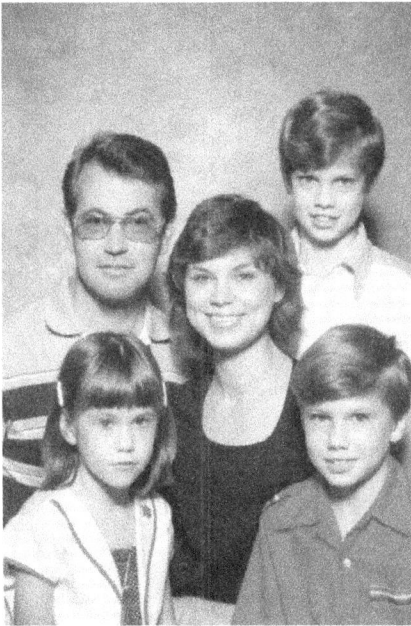

Family in 1983, while Linda was on kidney dialysis

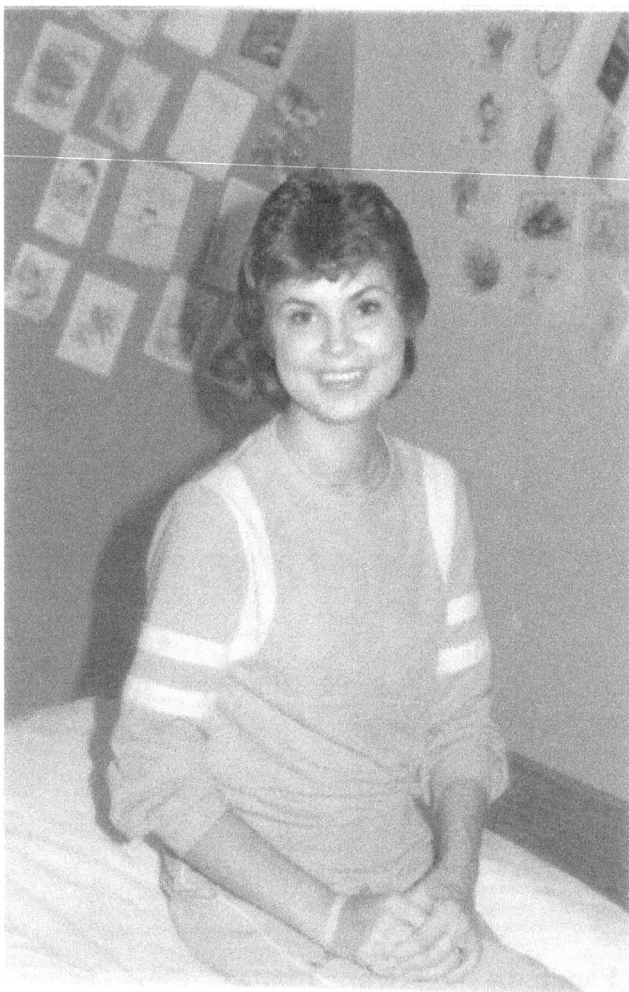

Linda in hospital after kidney transplant

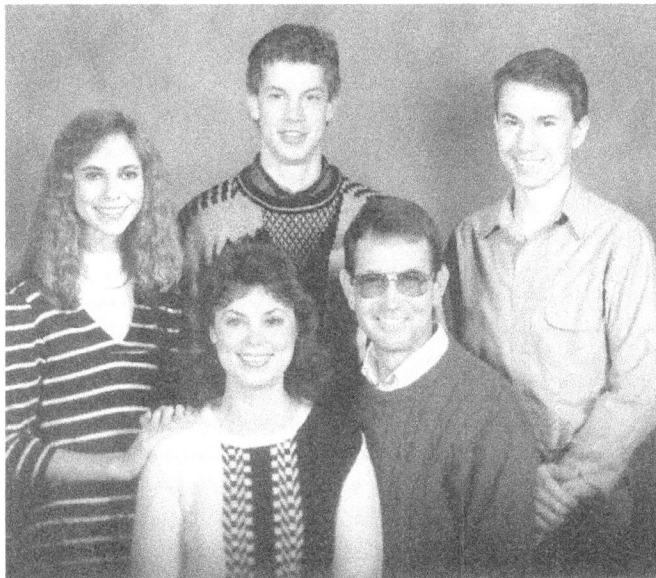

1994 Family Portrait

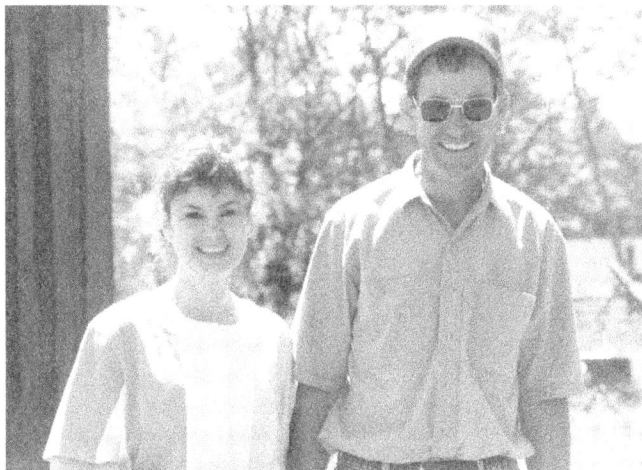

Linda and Aubin on Linda's Birthday in 1993

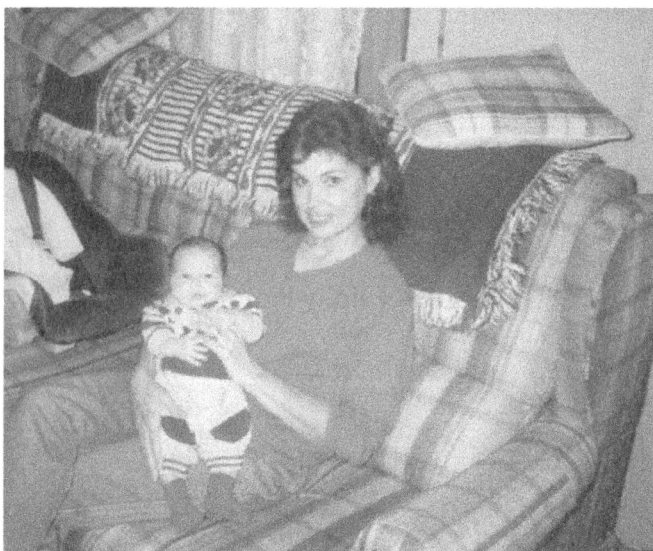

Linda in 1997, holding her first grandchild.

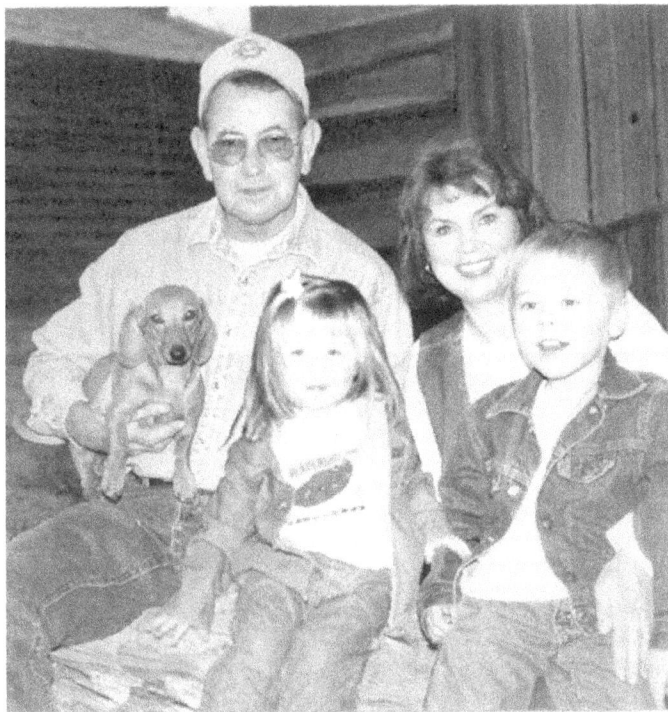

2001, Aubin and Linda with their grandchildren

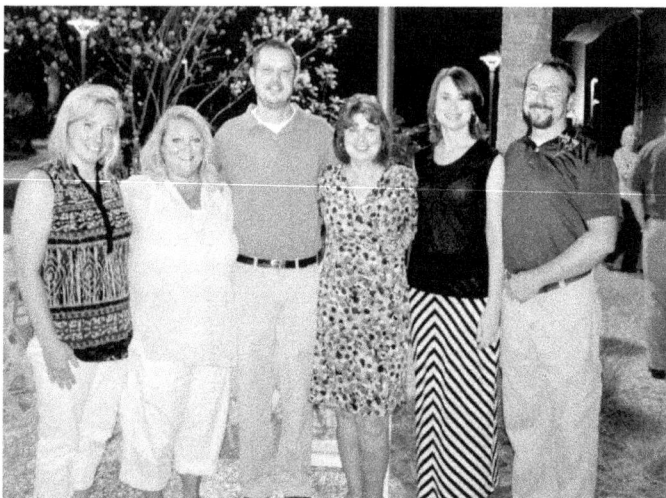

Linda with her grown children

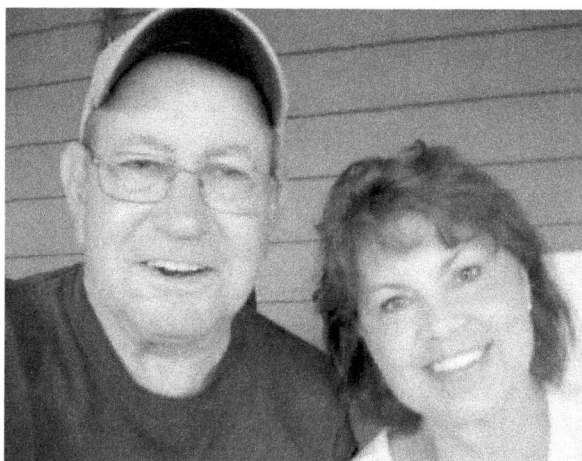

Aubin and Linda enjoying life on the Cumbie
Farm in Ephesus, Georgia.

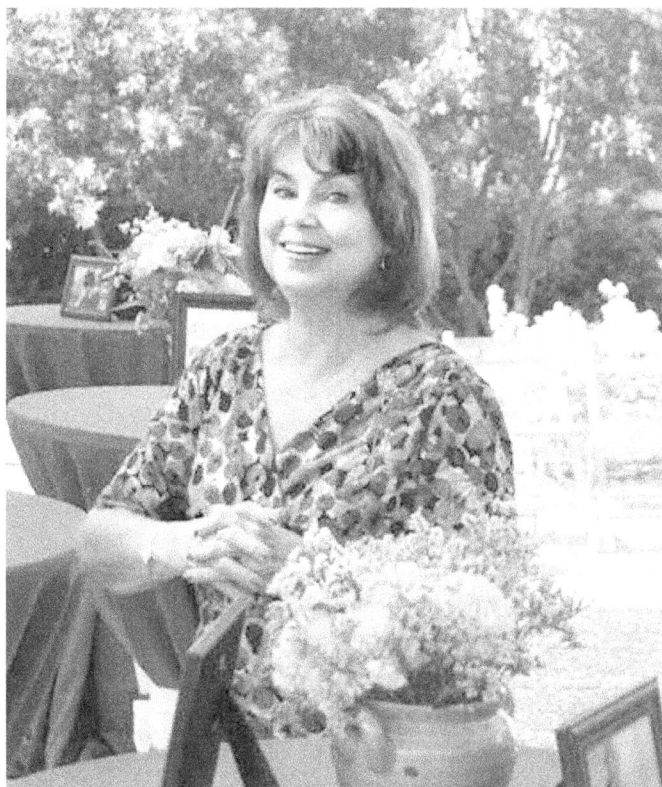

Linda today
Thirty-one years after receiving her kidney transplant.

Part 2: Daughter gives the Gift of Life to her Mother

Chapter 1 Emergency Hospital Visit

Sandra wasn't feeling her best as she headed to Ranburne Elementary School. She enjoyed working with the children; it was rewarding and gave her a sense of purpose. It provided her an opportunity to make a difference in the life of kids. It was April and the school year was quickly coming to an end with only a little over a month left before summer vacation. This time of year the children are thinking of everything, but school work and she knew how excited children get when the weather begins to get pretty outside.

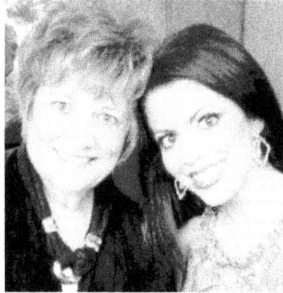

When she awoke that morning, she tried to shake the bad feeling she was having by eating breakfast. There was something going around at school and she wondered if she had caught it from one of the children in her class. She began to feel somewhat better as she dressed to go to school. Once she got to school the bad feeling returned and she became weak and faint. The school nurse realized something was wrong and called EMT to come quickly. When they arrived, they found Sandra conscious, but weak. She was admitted to Tanner Hospital for further tests to determine the problem. The test results indicated she had high levels of protein. She had been on blood pressure medicine for twenty-three years, but she had never felt quite like this before.

Chapter 2 Tragedy Strikes

Two days after Sandra went into the hospital her mother was admitted. She was placed on the same floor in the hospital as Sandra. She was there with her mother when she passed away in the hospital. During this trying time, Sandra found out she only had 13 percent kidney function in both kidneys. It was a difficult time for Sandra with the sudden loss of her mother and now having to deal with renal failure.

Chapter 3 Reflection of a Happy Family

During her hospital stay she had time to reflect on a time before she had children. Doctors had told her she would never have children. Her faith was strong and she decided to turn it over to God. Ten years later she gave birth to a son she named Jeremy. Sandra loved everything about being a mother. She had also prayed for a daughter with brown eyes and dark hair. She gave birth to a daughter named Mindy on February eighteenth. Mindy not only was born on the same date as Sandra, but they were born just two minutes apart at 7:40AM and 7:42AM. She now felt her family was complete.

Chapter 4 Mindy's Wish

Doctors predicted Sandra may only have six months before she would have to go on dialysis. Neither Jeremy nor Mindy wanted their mother to go on dialysis. While dialysis helps to buy time for those with renal failure, it is very limiting and diminishes the quality of life for the patient. Mindy felt dialysis was a lifesaver for people with renal failure, but it was only a bandage rather than a cure. She wanted to be the one to give Sandra a kidney.

Both Mindy and Jeremy had the "O" negative blood type like their mother. Mindy just knew she would be a perfect match. Jeremy agreed he would be there to give if Mindy was not a match.

Mindy and her mother were very close with so much in common. Both were left-handed. Both enjoyed singing together in church. Mindy found her mother's baptismal certificate, and discovered they both had been saved on an Easter Sunday, when they were both ten years old. The mother and daughter shared a strong bond of love.

Chapter 5 Reason for Renal Failure

There was concern that Sandra's condition was hereditary, and later Mindy could develop kidney disease. Mindy was a young mother with a beautiful little girl named Gracie. A young mother must also consider how donating a kidney will affect her when she has other children. Pregnancy and childbirth can sometimes take a toll on the mother's kidneys. The concerns are real for any family member facing kidney donation. After undergoing tests, the doctors contributed Sandra's renal failure to hypertension and not heredity. Mindy decided to go through with the donation.

Chapter 6 Time for a Transplant

By the end of July Sandra's kidney function had diminished to 9 percent. Without further treatment, she would have approximately six months of kidney function remaining. Mindy underwent a two-day process to determine her compatibility as a kidney donor.

On September 23 and 24 in 2010 Mindy reported to the Mason Transplant Center at Piedmont Hospital in Atlanta, Georgia. The tests showed she was a healthy candidate. The final test would count how many arteries were present on her kidneys. The test needed to show Mindy had one or two arteries on each side of the kidney. If there were three or four arteries, surgery would be risky. The tested indicated Mindy had two arteries on each kidney. She received a call from Leanne Whitehead Piedmont Hospital Living Donor Coordinator. Mindy was found to be a perfect match. She was overjoyed and thrilled to find out the news. According to

Mindy's research, each person who is born with two working kidneys has eight times the amount of kidney function needed in a lifetime. The kidney is very strong and with so many people who need a kidney she wished she had more kidneys to give.

Chapter 7 Kidney Transplant

Mindy and Sandra reported to Piedmont Hospital on Thursday for surgery scheduled the next day on November 19, 2010. Mindy would be giving a kidney to her mother. For Mindy and Sandra it was a time of mixed emotions. Sandra admired Mindy's courage and strength to willingly give a kidney. Sandra was concerned for her daughter and like any mother she did not want anything to happen to Mindy. She prayed God would continue to bless Mindy and find favor in her precious daughter.

Lying in her hospital bed the night before surgery, Sandra was reflecting on the time when she wanted to be a mother, but it had not seemed possible. Now the daughter she had prayed for was saving her. Sandra had such faith in God and she was thankful for such a Christian daughter.

The night before surgery Mindy had trouble sleeping. Everything was going through her mind. She was giving a gift of life to the one person who meant more to her than anyone in the world.

Sandra knew everything would go according to His plan for her life and Mindy was going to do just fine. After all they had so much in common. They both had faith in God and both knew with God all things are possible. (Matthew 19:26, KJV)

Chapter 8 Kidney Transplant Surgery

The night passed and the day of surgery arrived. Mindy and Sandra told each other how much they meant to each other trying not to cry. Mindy was filled with mixed emotions. She was filled with happiness, but she was also nervous about the outcome of the surgery. The last thought she had before she was given anesthesia was she may never awaken. She knew she would go to heaven, but she was not ready to leave Jerome, her husband, and Gracie, who was two years old. She was not ready to leave her family and friends. She knew it was in God's hands and she prayed His will be done.

Chapter 9 Surgery Recovery

After three hours of surgery, Sandra and Mindy were placed in separate rooms. Mindy was in the hospital for three days and Sandra remained for five days. Mindy could not wait to go see her mom for the first time knowing God healed her through her kidney. Sandra's body accepted the kidney without any complications. Before surgery Sandra had been fatigued and forgetful, but now she was full of energy. Sandra was no longer on a strict diet. After surgery she could eat the food she always enjoyed and drink juice instead of water. Sandra's recovery took three months. The medications had to be adjusted to prevent nausea. It usually takes longer for the kidney recipient to adjust to the antirejection drugs to prevent the body from rejecting the new kidney. She had to adjust to a new life.

Mindy had six weeks of recovery before getting back to work and her normal routine. Jerome, her husband, was so helpful during Mindy's surgery and recovery time. He was there to encourage Mindy from the very beginning when she decided to donate a kidney. Jerome supported her when she had to undergo the two-day evaluation process at Piedmont Hospital. He was there with her at every doctor's appointment. He took care of Gracie until Mindy was strong enough. He did all the cooking and cleaning, and drove Mindy back and forth to the doctor. They celebrated nine years of marriage in April. She felt blessed to have Jerome as her husband.

Chapter 10 Mindy's Testimony

The whole experience has humbled Mindy like never before.

Mindy attributes the success of the entire experience to her faith in God. Her hope is to tell her story so it will touch countless lives. She gives God all the Glory and she gives God all the praise for what He has done and continues to do in her life. She thanks God every day for healing her precious, beautiful, inspiring and, most of all, godly mother. "My mom gave me life. Now I am able to help sustain hers."

Mindy will continue to attend annual checkups to monitor the function of her remaining kidney. She knows God has a bigger plan for her life and she will remain healthy to fulfill His plan.

Author's Note

We met on a wet rainy day in a conference room where Mindy worked. Not knowing what to expect from the girl who had donated a kidney to her mother, I was curious. When she entered, her smile filled the room with light and without saying a word I knew she was more than someone who had donated a kidney to her mother. Other than being physically beautiful with big brown eyes and dark hair, there was so much more. She spoke softly about her experience and she radiated joy. She didn't have to tell me about her faith in God. It was obvious. She was kind and sweet and the more she talked I could see she just wanted to make sure I knew what God had done in her life. God had used her in a way to show others His love for all those who loved Him. She gave God all the glory and she wanted everyone to know God had been there with her each step of the way. She was not worried about the future. She knows God will take care of her and her family. Mindy is a walking testimony to what God can do. I will always remember the young mother who gave because as she said "It is more blessed to give than to receive." Acts 20:35

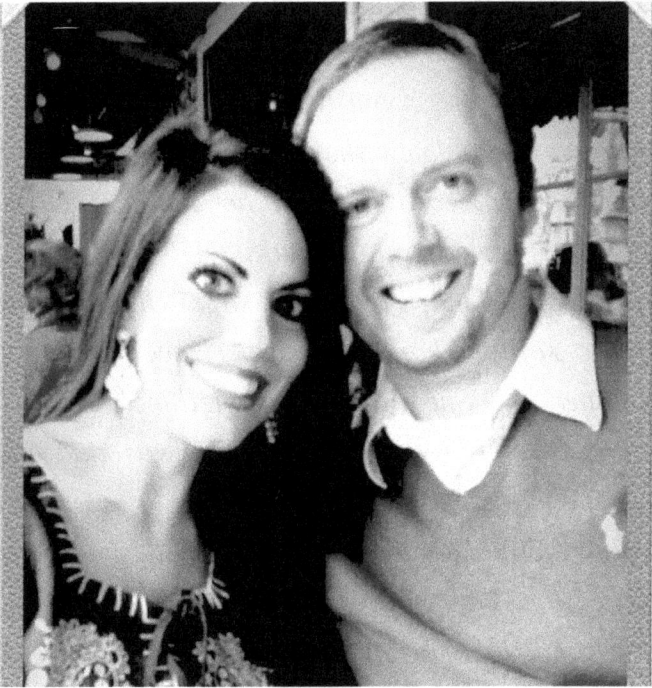

Mindy and Jerome, her husband

The Tale of Two Kidneys

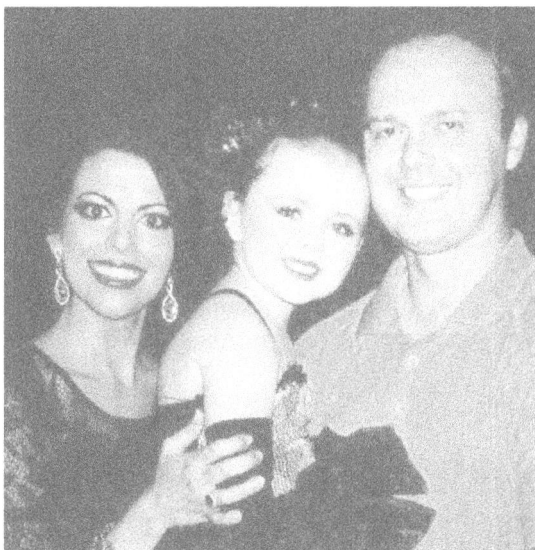

Mindy, Gracie, her daughter, and Jerome

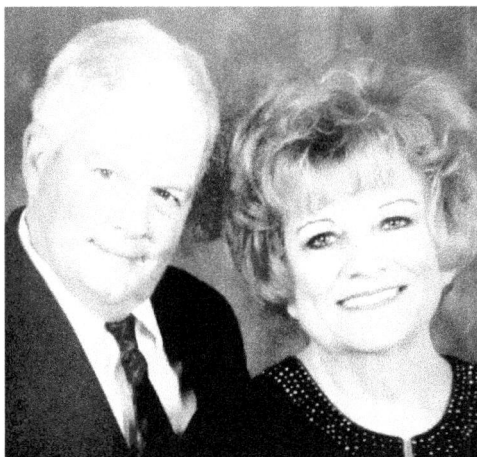

Danny and Sandra Harris

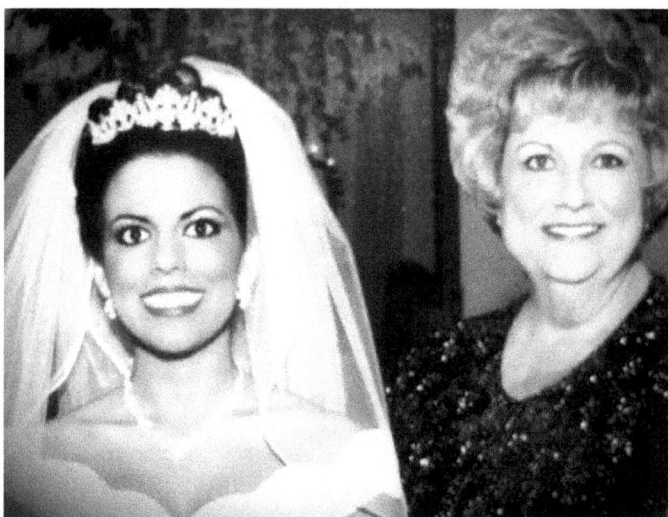

Mindy, on her wedding day, with Sandra

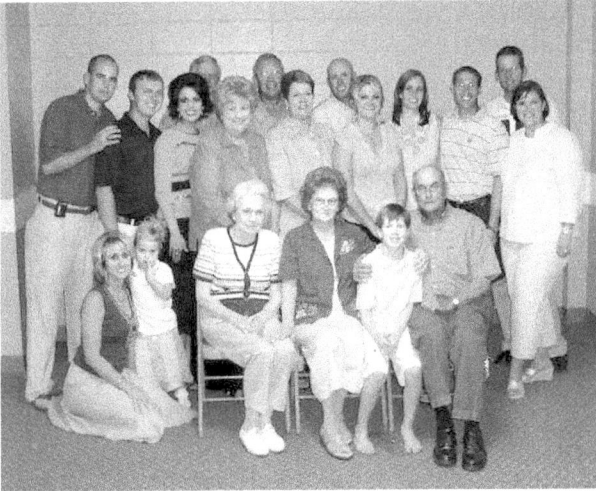

Mindy's family

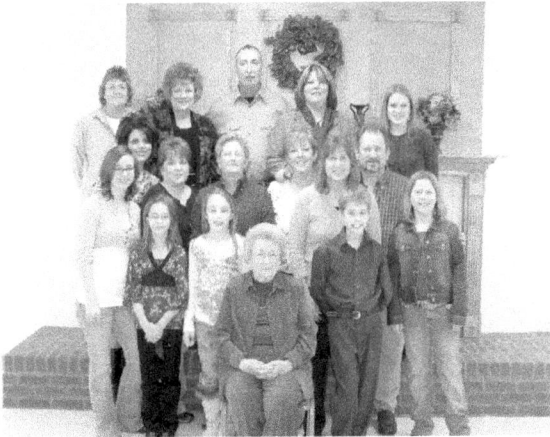

Mindy's family

Part 3 Donor Couples Donate Kidney to Each Other

The Tale of Two Kidneys

Let me share with you my tale of two kidneys. Richard, my husband, was on kidney dialysis for three years as a result of renal failure. He was becoming weaker and weaker and needed a kidney. We were not matches for each other, and neither were our daughters, Sam and Shea. I decided to donate my kidney to someone else to increase the odds of Richard receiving a kidney. Piedmont Hospital in Atlanta placed us on the Paired Kidney Donation program. The Paired Kidney Donation computerized network matches donors based on blood and tissue typing. Richard was matched to receive a kidney from Charlie, a high school teacher from Beavercreek High School in Ohio. Larry, Charlie's father, would receive my kidney. We began as total strangers and ended up as friends with a common purpose, to save the life of someone we loved.

Chapter 1 Richard and Renal Failure

During a sports physical examination when he was a freshman in college, the doctors discovered one of Richard's kidneys was smaller and not functioning and the other kidney was not filtering properly. He was not able to go out for football as he planned. Doctors told Richard to work at jobs where he could stay off his feet as much as possible. Richard's idea was to work as hard as he could for as long as he could. He was determined to live life to the fullest and to continue to do the things he enjoyed. He was very strong-willed. All he had to hear was "you can't do that," and he would work so much harder to prove he could do whatever he set his mind to do. He worked hard and never complained.

Fifty years later he received news from Dr. Fredrickson, his nephrologist, that his kidney function was diminishing and he would have to begin kidney dialysis. It was nearing the end of

June and we had planned a family get-together at the lake for the 4th of July. This holiday was one of our family's favorite times of year. We always loved everything about the 4th of July. This year proved to be extra special. We had invited Richard's brothers and their families to the lake. Robin, my brother, Mom, her sister and her family were going to be there. Richard asked the doctor if he could wait until after the 4th. Reluctantly he explained the seriousness of the situation to Richard. There was a chance Richard could become sick and need to undergo emergency dialysis treatment. He did explain to Richard it was not ideal and there was a risk in waiting. Richard decided to wait until after the 4th to report to the hospital to have a port placed in his stomach.

We had planned a Barbeque with hamburgers, hot dogs, and all the trimmings. Watermelon and Shea's famous Flag Cake rounded off the menu. The sun did seem brighter and warmer than usual. The sun rays danced on the water like crystals making it the prettiest 4th of July ever. Everyone went swimming, boat riding and skiing. We played croquet on the lawn. Mom always enjoyed playing and beating everyone. Firing up the grill with the smell of hamburgers and hotdogs gave the men a chance to show off their cooking skills.

Fireworks were planned for the evening. Richard and Shea loved stopping by the Fireworks Store each year to get the latest new and improved fireworks. Richard, Robin and Shea were in charge of the fireworks show. As I watched the sun go down everyone in lawn chairs began watching the fireworks light up the sky over the water. No matter how many fireworks you have, there are never enough. It was a wonderful time with family making memories we would hold dear for a long time.

Richard water skied and he was better than ever. He knew once he started dialysis he would no longer be allowed to swim in the lake for fear of getting infections from lake water. Looking back at pictures, we realized Richard was very sick. His skin was turning gray and he looked very tired. Richard was now ready for whatever lay ahead.

On July 11, he reported to the hospital to have the port placed in his stomach to begin the process of kidney dialysis. It was performed as outpatient surgery and afterwards we headed home. It would be two weeks before he would begin dialysis. He discussed his treatment options with the doctor to have peritoneal dialysis which could be performed at home or to have hemodialysis, which is done at a center away from home. Both have their advantages and disadvantages. It was a personal choice of each patient and their physician.

Chapter 2 Peritoneal Dialysis, or PD

Richard and Dr. Fredrickson decided peritoneal dialysis or PD would be the best solution for treatment. Peritoneal dialysis can be done in the privacy of your home. We reported to the clinic for training in how to properly do PD.

Richard quickly learned the steps to perform PD. Everyone at the clinic was so nice and willing to help. The doctor and nurses were upbeat and this made the training easier. The first step was for Richard to learn to do manual exchanges. Once Richard received training on the cycler machine, he was given the machine to take home. Richard would be attached to the cycler by a tube with a catheter placed in the peritoneum in his stomach. His PD schedule was for eight continual hours on the cycler machine each night. He was able to sleep during the exchange, but he had to be extremely careful to make sure everything was sterile to cut down on germs, bacteria and infections.

After he completed each exchange, he would get supplies ready for the next exchange. They increase the amount of time to an extra manual exchange in the middle of the day. The first year Richard worked four hours each day. His work schedule allowed him to finish work and return home to do a manual exchange. We were settling into a routine of kidney dialysis. The machine was quiet and sleeping was not a problem. Richard continued to get up and down during most nights. Leg cramps were a problem and, most of the time, the last exchange on the cycler seemed to pull on the inside of his stomach. It would wake him and he would get up and sit in a chair until it was finished.

For the next three years we continued living life trying not to let PD dictate how we were going to live.   Dr. Frederickson knew patients who had been on dialysis for more than twenty-five years. This eased our minds, knowing there were patients who were successfully on kidney dialysis. Being able to do dialysis at home seemed to work well with few problems.

Chapter 3 Challenges Faced on Dialysis

During the PD training, the nurse stressed the importance of sterilizing the catheter and maintaining a germ free environment. Masks were worn during the exchanges to avoid contracting an infection. Peritonitis is the most common infection for PD patients. Richard was to take his temperature every morning. Right after he started PD his fever escalated to 102^0. We called the doctor and he wanted him to report to the emergency room immediately. When we arrived at the emergency room, his temperature was 103.5^0. Dr. Fredrickson had called ahead and they were expecting him. They brought his fever down and ran tests to see if he had an infection. Richard spent a night in the hospital, but the tests did not indicate an infection. They did not discover why his fever went up so high. Richard's temperature remained constant for the remainder of the time he was on PD. He was not hospitalized any more while on dialysis.

The company which delivered the dialysis supplies to our home would also deliver supplies anywhere we requested in the United States. All we had to do was to give them prior notice of the date and place to deliver. We decided to give it a try, and go on a vacation.

The first trip was to go to Washington, D.C., and to tour the Capitol. We ordered the dialysis solution to be sent to the hotel where we would be staying. On the trip we decided not to take the cycler and do manual exchanges for the week we were there. He would do three exchanges during the day and one right before bedtime. The manual exchanges did not filter as well as the machine and he retained more fluid than usual in his legs, ankles and feet. He never complained, but I could tell he was uncomfortable. The company delivered the supplies we had requested. When we arrived at the hotel there were fifteen big boxes of solution behind the registration desk. They delivered the boxes to our room without any questions.

The Tale of Two Kidneys

Apparently other kidney dialysis patients had stayed in their hotel. When you are on dialysis, you feel you are the only person on dialysis. It was a great trip to our capital and we were able to visit the White House and go on several tours. The trip was successful and we returned home with a renewed sense of freedom. We thought we had mastered dialysis while traveling on trips.

We planned another trip to Las Vegas, Nevada. We planned to fly out and rent a car to visit Hoover Dam and other sights. We ordered the supplies we would need for four days. Before leaving, we received confirmation the supplies had been delivered to the hotel. We knew how long the flight from Atlanta to Las Vegas would be, but we had not calculated the extra time in the airports. The arrival time to the hotel made for a long day. Richard had missed his midday exchange and his legs were beginning to swell.

When we arrived at the hotel, they did not have any record of the supplies arriving. It was on a Saturday afternoon and the supply company was closed for the weekend. The next flight home would be the following day. It was a helpless feeling not knowing who to call. The employee over the supply room had looked several times and checked the computer and it was as if the supplies had vanished. By now I was beginning to panic and I started to cry. People standing around were coming up and patting me on the shoulder.

The employee was doing all she could do to find the supplies. How hard could it be to find fifteen big boxes in a supply room? The boxes had been delivered. She finally asked me to come and see if I could help her locate the boxes. We were staying in the MGM Hotel. When I entered the supply area, it was as big as a city block. Their supply area was bigger than most hotels. Now I understood why she was having such a hard time locating the boxes. It was like finding a needle in a haystack. She decided to check the computer one last time for the supplies. She found the supplies had been filed under Richard's first name "R" instead of his last name "C."

We placed the boxes on a cart and she took them to our room using the service elevators. She was so nice and patient and she had continued looking for the boxes until they were found. I had become a number one basket case. I was now crying out of joy because the supplies had been found. I knew she was relieved to find the supplies so she could get rid of me. The rest of the trip I looked for her to tell her thanks, but I never saw her again. Something just told me she probably saw me coming and hid. I hope she did not quit, because every hotel needs an employee like her. The rest of the trip went smoothly and we had a wonderful time. We proved to ourselves traveling while on dialysis could be done.

Preparing the solution for the exchanges on trips could be done with planning ahead of time. The solution needed to be warmed to room temperature before it could be used. We traveled with a heating pad to warm the solution bag to room temperature. Once in a while the heating pad would get it too hot and he would have to wait until it cooled down. The clinic staff did not recommend using a microwave because the bag could overheat. While traveling in a car, the bag of solution could be placed on the dash of the car to let the sun warm it.

We decided to go on our annual camping trip at Port Saint Joe, Florida on the Gulf. Packing the camper with enough supplies for a week felt more like we were moving away. We had boxes of supplies everywhere. Everything went smoothly until we were packing up to come home. Richard got ready to connect the camper to the truck, but he did not have the strength to manually connect the hitch of the camper to the truck. He had always been able to do it before without any problems. Everyone in our group had left. He stopped and rested. After an hour he tried again and was able to connect the camper to the truck. When we returned, we had an automatic hitch installed on the camper thus solving the problem. It had been another great trip. We were little by little becoming experienced at traveling while on kidney dialysis.

We planned to go to Birmingham for a New Year's Eve Dance and celebration. We had traveled to the lake house to get ready and planned to come back after the dance and stay for a few days. As we were leaving, I looked and Richard's white shirt was red with blood. The blood was coming from the catheter. We immediately packed up and quickly headed home arriving home after midnight. We did everything we knew to get the bleeding to stop, but were not successful. The emergency phone operator remained calm and was able to tell us what to do to stop the bleeding. Early morning around 3:00 A.M., everything settled down and we were able to get some rest. A nervous way to end the year with the onset of a fresh new year. We anticipated a great new year ahead and hoped to find a kidney donor.

Kidney patients on PD are always aware of the weather. In the three years he was on dialysis there were several threats of severe weather, thunderstorms and a chance of tornadoes headed in our direction. Connected to a machine, with the threat of tornadoes, was unnerving. We decided to move everything down to the lower level of our home and sleep there for the night. We always watched the weather report before going to bed to make sure bad weather was not going to move into our area in the middle of the night. Loss of electricity in our area was also a concern. We were fortunate to have this happen only once and the power company worked to return power as soon as possible.

All computerized machines have the ability to malfunction and the cycler machine was no different. Since the machine was used at night, the machine would malfunction in the middle of the exchange or around 11:30pm. The number to call for assistance was helpful and the operators could walk you through steps to correct the problem. Most of the operators we talked with lived on the west coast which meant they were several hours behind us and not as sleepy. Once they could not repair the machine over the phone and it had to be replaced. The company provided 24-hour service and we received another cycler the next day.

Another challenge was ordering the correct amount of supplies for a month. Seems easy enough, but trying to keep it accurate was not as easy as you might think. There were different size bags with different strengths to the solutions. There were different solution bags for the cycler machine and different bags for manual exchanges. The order was placed during the middle of each month for the next month. The size and strengths of the bags were never the same from month to month. Richard would go to the clinic for monthly checkups and they would change the size of bags or strengths. It would be at least three weeks before supplies would be delivered. There were other supplies which were ordered such as the tubing and connectors for each exchange. Planning a month ahead was tricky.

It was a challenge storing a month of supplies. We would receive forty big boxes each month. Taking inventory and keeping up with everything was mind boggling. One room in the basement was used to store the supplies for a month. Walking the supplies up from the basement to our bedroom was done twice a day.

The room used to do exchanges had to be sterile. Extra precautions were taken to make sure bacteria was not present during the exchanges. Masks were worn by everyone present during an exchange. The room was closed off during exchanges.

Three years on dialysis went by quickly. Richard had a routine he followed. We had settled into a daily schedule working around the PD schedule. Dialysis was doing the job of his kidney by keeping him alive. Dialysis was a blessing, and we were thankful it was available. At our fingertips were people we could call if there was a problem or concern. We met incredible people at the hospital and in the clinics, who were concerned about your well-being. The challenges along the way were just that and nothing more. Keeping a positive attitude helped to keep everything in perspective.

Chapter 4 Three Years of Dialysis

It appeared dialysis was going to be a part of our lives forever. Each year we would report to the transplant center for reevaluation. The first Living Donor coordinator assigned to me was not very encouraging. One day he called to tell me I was not a match for Richard. During the call he informed me we would never find another Paired Donor couple. I knew we did not have the same blood type, but my hope was to find a Paired Donor couple. Richard had "O" type blood which meant he could give to anyone, but he could only receive a kidney from someone with "O" type. My blood type was "A" which meant I could only be a match to donate a kidney to a person with "A" type blood. Any couple that was in the reverse situation would be able to give to each other and they would not need my kidney. This meant the odds that Richard and I would find another couple looked impossible. The coordinator told me not to get my hopes up, since he had never heard it happening before. He meant well, but I did not want to hear it was impossible. I dismissed the thought, choosing to believe there was a couple out there.

Chapter 5 The Wait for a Kidney Donor

For two years we continued to go to the yearly evaluations. During the second year evaluation, Piedmont Hospital Living Donor Coordinator, Leanne Whitehead, offered us hope we would find a couple. After our yearly evaluation we were preparing to leave and she quietly said the doctors were working to find a match for Richard to receive a kidney. This gave us a glimmer of hope to know they had not forgotten about us. We had friends which were tested to see if they were matches for Richard. Even though they did not match for various reasons, it helped to know they were willing to donate a kidney. Our sister-in-law, Sheila, would call Richard to let him know she was trying to find him a kidney. Her calls seem to come at times when he was feeling his lowest. Those calls always made him feel better and helped to keep his spirits up. He received cards of encouragement from family and friends. It did not take much to keep hope alive during those years on dialysis.

Chapter 6 The Impossible became Possible

On April 11, just when it looked as if nothing was happening, I received a call from Leanne. They had found a couple for us. It was on a Friday afternoon and she wanted me come to the hospital for further tests to see if I was a match. The tests would also determine if I was healthy enough to donate a kidney.

The nurses and hospital staff administering the test were cheering me on with each test. The tread mill test, I thought, would be easy, turned out to be harder than I thought. On the treadmill at home I could walk thirty minutes or three miles whichever came first. She asked me if I thought I could stay on the treadmill for nine minutes. Not to brag, but I told her, "No problem." Walking on their treadmill was so different for the test. Before the nine minutes were up, the treadmill was inclined to the equivalent of climbing Mt. Everest or so it seemed. The speed was increased and I was running as fast as I could, hanging onto the arm rest. She was laughing at me as I neared the nine minute mark. There I was running all bent over, with my tongue hanging out before I finished. When she said nine minutes were up, I gladly stopped. I passed the tread mill test!

Another test performed was the Glo-Fil test to check my kidney function. You drink a liter of water every ten minutes for an hour. They check your output every 15 minutes. Everything went well, but on the way home at the end of the day I was stopping at every convenience store to go to the restroom for the fifty-mile ride home. It was two intense days of testing and I passed.

Chapter 7 The Paired Donor Couple

The person who would receive my kidney was Larry and he was the same age as Richard. He had "A" blood type. Charlie was Larry's son and he was a match for Richard with "O" type blood. Charlie had planned to donate a kidney to his dad. From my understanding, his dad received a blood transfusion leaving him with antibodies. Father and son were no longer perfect matches for each other. Larry and I were perfect matches. The first coordinator meant well, but he was wrong. A paired donor couple had been found. Kidney donors go to where the kidney recipient is located. I was to go to Miami Valley Hospital in Dayton, Ohio. Charlie was to come to Atlanta at Piedmont Hospital to give to Richard.

Chapter 8 The Journey to Dayton Ohio

As I woke, from a seemingly sleepless night, it dawned on me I was 500 miles away from home in a place I would never have imagined. The day before, I had left Richard, Sam and Shea, in Georgia to fly to Dayton, Ohio. I had waited until the day before surgery to leave. Secretly I was afraid something might go wrong and the surgery would be canceled. Richard was getting weaker and weaker on dialysis and I feared he might not be able to last until a donor was found. There were some blood tests I would have to undergo when I arrived in Ohio. The staff at Miami Valley Hospital had never met me and they insisted I have the final blood tests completed at their hospital before surgery. I tried to reassure myself the tests were going to be fine. Piedmont Hospital had performed all the tests and the results were sent to the hospital. The test results showed I was a perfect match for the man who would receive my kidney. Everything seemed so strange and different in a place where the only person I knew was my brother, Robin. He had insisted on going with me and I was relieved. He had to make plans to take off from work to travel with me. For the past three months, it seemed like everyone was having to change their schedules for us.

The sun was just coming up when we arrived at the hospital at 6:30am on Wednesday, July 6, 2011. You could tell it was going to be a beautiful summer day.

As we entered and looked around the waiting room, we saw families with small children. A few couples were talking to each other. They were waiting with someone who was also going to have surgery. It was early and everyone seemed rested. The whole time I wanted to tell them what was going on and what was about to happen. Feeling apprehensive about the surgery, I just wanted it to be over.

They wasted no time preparing me for surgery. The small room was filled with doctors, nurses and medical staff. There was an air of excitement and urgency among the staff, with everyone performing a specific task. Finally I could breathe a sigh of relief knowing the day had arrived and they were going to operate. It had been a long three months waiting for the surgery to be scheduled. Later I would learn that this was the first Paired Donor kidney donor transplant for Miami Valley Hospital. Everything had to be coordinated between two hospitals in different states. Piedmont Hospital had found a couple to match us at Miami Valley Hospital. Robin was concerned about my well-being and he was standing by my bed talking to the doctors and staff. I smiled when someone thought Robin was the doctor who would be performing the surgery. The surgeon entered the small room and with a black marker placed a letter "L" on my stomach. He planned to remove my left kidney.

By the end of the day I would experience one of the greatest miracles of my life.

The IV in my hand quickly put me into a deep sleep.

Chapter 9 The Day before Surgery

Ann Taylor, the Living Donor Coordinator, greeted me with a basket of flowers and a big smile when we arrived at the Dayton Airport. Robin and I were to go to the hospital as soon as possible. We had left around 4:00 A.M., headed to the Hartsfield-Jackson Atlanta International Airport. I was not supposed to eat anything before the final blood test. Eating ice chips all the way kept me busy on the plane ride to Dayton. By the time I arrived at Miami Valley Hospital I was a mess. I felt and looked like something the cat had drugged in from outside. When we arrived at the hospital, I had to stop and take a minute to freshen up in the hospital's public restroom. No matter what I did I looked tired and it showed. It seemed the harder I tried to go fast, the slower I was moving. Robin was telling me I looked great, but that is what a good brother does when his sister needs some encouragement. Besides he looked fresh, smiling and talking to everyone. He was so charming and I was so tired, nervous and a little scared about what was going to happen to all four of the participants.

Chapter 10 Press Conference

A press conference was scheduled as soon as we arrived. When we walked in there were news reporters, hospital staff and Larry, the kidney recipient, who would be receiving my kidney. He was there with Christa, his wife,- and members of his family. They made us feel like we were a part of their family. The room was filled to standing room only. You could feel the excitement of the event which was going to take place. They asked me questions about the Paired Donor program and I was trying so hard to answer the questions. The only thing I knew was my name and my brother's name. Everything else I babbled away sounding more like I did not know anything, but my brother Robin was there and he took over and calmly answered most of the questions. I had worked myself into a nervous frenzy while at the same time trying to act like it was just another day.

I was looking forward to meeting Larry. Richard and his story were similar and both had

115

been on dialysis for a while. Christa was so nice and easy to talk too. She immediately put me at ease and I could feel myself relaxing. Their son, Charlie, was in Atlanta at Piedmont Hospital ready to donate a kidney to Richard. It must have been hard on Christa, but it did not show. Both her husband and son were having surgery. Up until I met her, I had not thought about the full impact kidney transplants have on the families involved. When you donate a kidney you are impacting the life of all the family members. I was feeling responsible for the kidney Larry was going to receive. I so wanted my kidney to work for him. This whole time I had spent my time and concentrated efforts on Richard receiving a kidney. The final outcome for us was in God's hands.

After the conference, there was a time for pictures and talking to Larry and Christa. Around 4:00 p.m., I met with Dr. Erik Weise, the surgeon who would be performing my surgery. He told me what to expect and he answered all my questions. The surgery would be done laparoscopically with a small robotic mechanical claw. A small incision would be made to remove the kidney. Surgery time for the donor is less invasive and recovery time shortened.

Chapter 11 Day of Surgery

Richard reported to Piedmont Hospital the morning of surgery. Sam and Shea would stay with their dad in Atlanta. Our friends, family and pastor came to the hospital to provide moral support to Richard. Larry reported to the hospital after I arrived. The donor's kidney is removed first and prepared for the kidney recipient. The hospitals work closely together making sure both donors are under anesthesia before continuing with surgery. A call is made to notify the other hospital to continue with the plans of removing the kidney. It was explained to me that Charlie and I could decide not to go through with donating our kidneys and just tell them we changed our minds. The recipients would not be told the reason the surgery was called off.

Charlie came to Atlanta with his wife Jenny a few days earlier. They went to an Atlanta Braves Baseball Game and were able to visit some of the sights around town before the day of surgery. Charlie was in his forties. He looked so young and healthy. He was strong and in great shape. He was our only hope of receiving a kidney. There were not any words to describe how grateful we were to him.

Chapter 12 The Day was Indeed Beautiful

The day ended as I had hoped. When I opened my eyes, Robin was telling me the wonderful news about Richard. The kidney he received began working immediately while he still was on the operating table. It is not unusual for it to take a few days before the new kidney begins working. Larry received my kidney and seemed to be doing well. It takes a longer recovery period for those who receive a kidney.

Chapter 13 Recovery

Everyone who has donated a kidney has a unique story. For me surgery was on a Wednesday. I was released from the hospital on Thursday morning. We were 500 miles away from home, so Robin and I made the most of the day by going to a movie and some yard sales.

Friday morning Robin and I went back to see Larry who was recovering in the hospital. He looked great and we talked about the experience. I would be leaving Dayton early Saturday morning and I would not see him again. His beautiful wife and I became friends on Facebook™.

Robin and I went to another movie on Friday afternoon. Saturday morning we headed to the airport for our flight back to Atlanta. I was carrying my basket of flowers I had received when we arrived. We arrived in Atlanta and I headed to Piedmont Hospital to see Richard. When I got off the elevator, Richard was walking down the hall to greet me. Sam went back to her home, and I spent the night in a foldout chair in Richard's hospital room. It was the best sleep just knowing everyone was doing well and we made it. On Sunday I met Charlie and Jenny, his wife, they were preparing to go home to Ohio.

Richard was dismissed from Piedmont on Sunday afternoon. Richard reported back to Mason Transplant Center at Piedmont Hospital three times a week for the first month. Sam lived near the hospital and she invited us to come and stay with her. We would stop by to see her, rest up and head home. Richard's checkups were reduced to twice a week for the second month. Each month it became easier to go for checkups. His new kidney was doing well and he was tolerating the medicine.

This year marks our Third year Anniversary. Richard's new kidney is working well. My health after donating a kidney is excellent and I have been dismissed.

Chapter 14 God's Perfect Plan

God had orchestrated each step of His plan and it was perfect. There were so many things which had to occur in order for our surgery to happen. My age was a concern for me. In some states and in many foreign countries donors must be under the age of 59 to be considered. When I signed up to be a donor, I was 58 years old. When I turned sixty, Richard was on dialysis and we did not have a donor. If a Paired Donor couple was located would I still be healthy enough to donate a kidney? Once a couple was located again there were some things which needed to be resolved in order to proceed with the Paired Donor surgery.

Miami Valley Hospital would only perform the surgery on a Wednesday. Piedmont Hospital performs transplant surgery only on Fridays. The surgeon at Miami Valley had conflicts with his schedule and the only time they could do the surgery was July 6. Piedmont changed their schedule to accommodate Miami Valley Hospital. The week of July 4th is an extremely busy time for surgeries. Leanne called me to let me know when they had scheduled the surgery. She knew how difficult it was going to be to get a surgery room on a Wednesday. She sounded a little worried about being able to secure the surgery rooms. If the previous Living Donor Coordinator had still been on staff, would he have tried to get the surgery scheduled? He never thought we would find a couple. It was now in Leanne's hands to coordinate our surgery with Piedmont and an out-of-state hospital. She was committed to getting the surgery date scheduled. Two years after the transplant Miami Valley Hospital informed me they had discontinued performing Paired Donor kidney transplants. The reason was unknown, but there was a small window of time they were there for Larry and me to have the surgery. Everything seemed to fall into place in God's Perfect Plan.

That day my life changed forever and I will never be the same. Yes, it was a beautiful day and every day since has been beautiful.

For we know that for those who love God all things work together for good, for those who are called according to his purpose. Romans 8:28

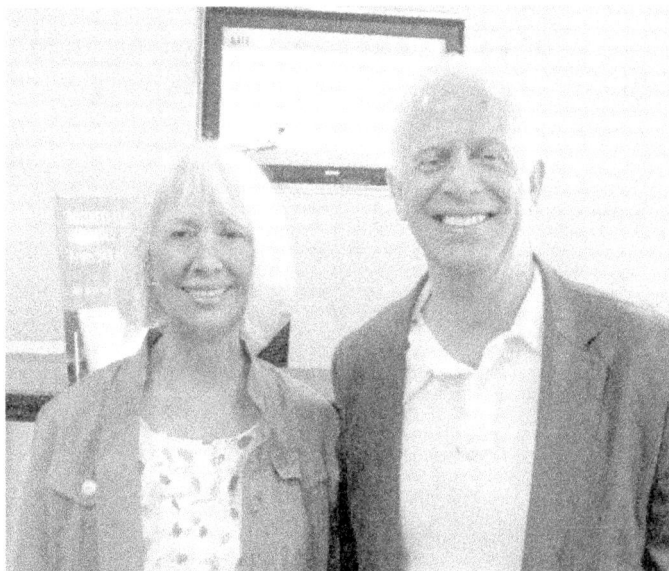

Robin and Becky at Atlanta Airport leaving for Dayton, Ohio on July 5, 2011

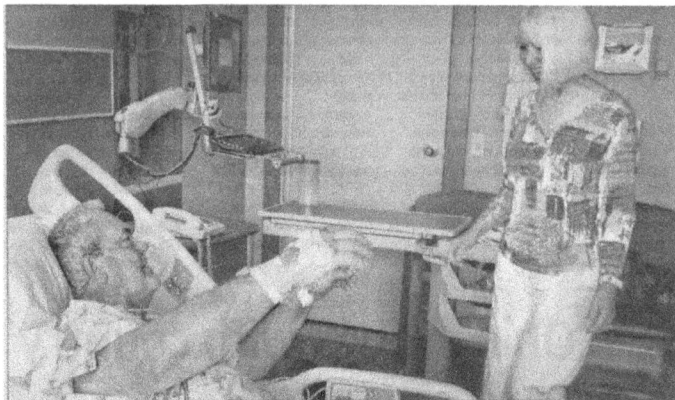

Larry on Friday, July 8, 2011, recovering from surgery and greeting Becky before she leaves to come home.

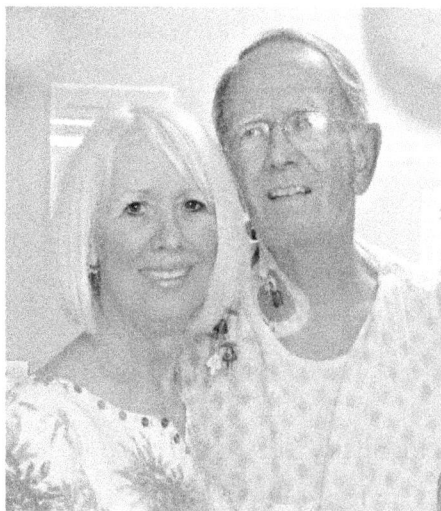

Saturday, July 9, 2011 Becky back in Atlanta, Georgia with Richard at Piedmont Hospital.

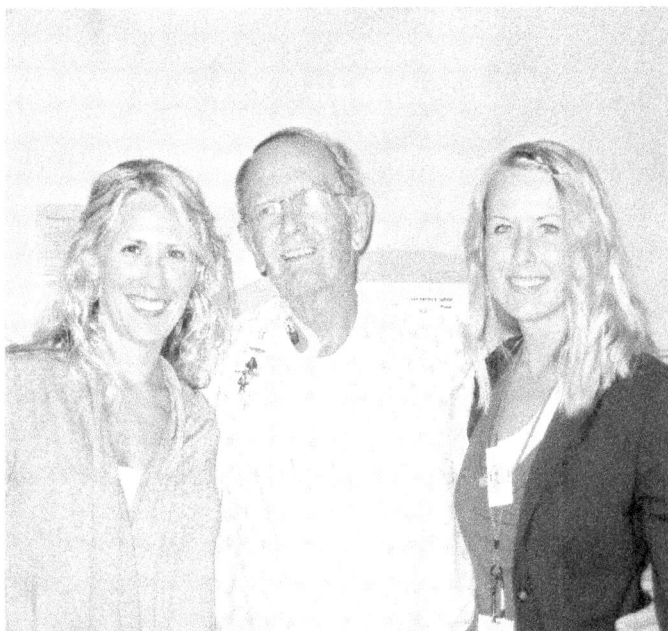

Sam and Shea with Richard at Piedmont Hospital
2 days after surgery

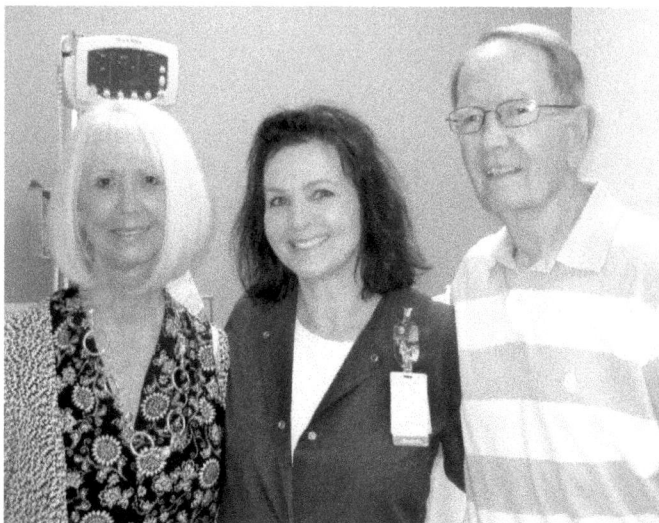

April 2014, Richard and Becky completed their
third year check up with Mason Transplant
Center at Piedmont Hospital. It's been three years
since Richard received a kidney. It's time to
celebrate. Pictured with them is Leanne
Whitehead, the Living Donor Coordinator.

Part 4
Kidney
Donation

Chapter 1 Being a Living Kidney Donor

More than 90,000 people in the United States are waiting for a kidney transplant. Every day, about eighteen people waiting will lose their lives before getting a new kidney.

There are new procedures which provide minimally invasive surgeries. Removing the kidney robotically produces better results. Patients have experienced faster recovery with less pain and discomfort and fewer visible scars. The new surgical procedure allows the doctors to remove a kidney using smaller incisions than ever before. Today the living donors are usually out of the hospital within two days, and back at work within a minimum of two weeks.[3]

Living donors can be siblings, parents, relatives, friends, in-laws, neighbors, co-workers,

---

[3]   Found   at   http://www.piedmont.org. Accessed 5/3/2014

religious service members, and even altruistic strangers. There are a few requirements that must be met for living donation.

- Good physical and mental health
- Must be at least 18 years old
- Must have a body mass index (BMI) that is less than 35
- Must be free from the following:
  - Uncontrolled high blood pressure
  - Diabetes
  - Cancer
  - HIV/AIDS
  - Hepatitis
  - Organ diseases
  - Infectious diseases[4]

If you meet the criteria and are interested in becoming a live kidney donor contact Piedmont Hospital, Mason Transplant Center in Atlanta, Georgia.

---

[4] Found at: http://www.hopsonsmedicine.org Accessed 5/31/2014

Chapter 2 Even in Death You can make a Difference

Donation after Death

It is also very important that potential donors make their wishes known. While many donors give a kidney to a friend or family member in need, kidneys harvested after death are the most common. If you have hesitated to sign a donor card because you feel your organs may not be suitable due to health problems or your age, you can now consider doing it. Be sure to tell your loved ones about your intentions to donate your organs after you die. Consent will need to be given by your next of kin before any organs are removed after death. As the time for viability of organs after death is limited, it is important to have your wishes known and understood.[5]

---

[5] Found at: http://seniorhealth.about.com Accessed 5/31/2014

Living Will

A Living Will, also called a Health Care Directive, specifies whether you would like to be kept on artificial life support if you become permanently unconscious or are otherwise dying and unable to speak for yourself. This can be done without an attorney. Free printable Living Wills are online customized to a specific state. Print and sign the Living Will. Specify your wishes to have your organs donated. Tell your family of your wishes.[6]

"It is a far, far better thing that I do, than I have ever done; it is a far, far better rest that I go to than I have ever known." <u>The Tale of Two Cities,</u> (Charles Dickens, 1859) is full of hope.

<u>Sharing Lives: A Tale of Two Kidneys</u> is also filled with hope for all those in need of a kidney. There is renewed awareness for healthy people to come forward and donate a kidney to a family member, a friend or a stranger and for everyone to become an organ donor either in life or death. Out of the ashes of grief rise hope and a better life for someone.

BIBLIOGRAPHY

CMV, http://health.ny.gov . April, 2014.

Dickens, Charles. A Tale of Two Cities. London: Chapman and Hall. 1859.

http://www.hopsonsmedicine.org Accessed 5/31/2014.

http://www.piedmont.org.   Accessed 5/3/2014.

http://seniorhealth.about.com. Accessed 5/31/2014.

http://www.totallegal.com. Accessed 5/30/2014.

Urine tests.   www.nih.gov. May 2014.

About the Author

Rebecca Carlisle lives in Roopville, Georgia, with her husband, Richard.

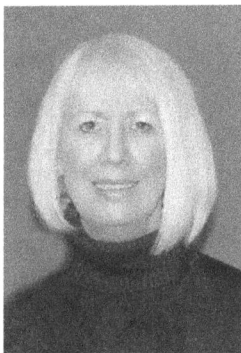

Ending her forty-year career in education as Principal of Ephesus Elementary School, she is now enjoying her retirement. She enjoys traveling, camping and working in the garden. She loves living in the country with her five cats and her dog, named Buckley. She has two daughters, who live close enough to visit often. Since retiring, she has written articles for Lifetouch and Christian Focus Publishers. Her first book, 52 Hats: A Memoir, is a story about her Christian mother.